Maria Clara Santos Araújo
Antonio da Costa Cardoso Neto
Márcia Silva de Oliveira

BREASTFEEDING

Maria Clara Santos Araújo
Antonio da Costa Cardoso Neto
Márcia Silva de Oliveira

BREASTFEEDING

Nursing Care

ScienciaScripts

Imprint

Cover image: www.ingimage.com

This book is a translation from the original published under ISBN 978-613-9-62643-4.

Publisher:
Sciencia Scripts
is a trademark of
Dodo Books Indian Ocean Ltd. and OmniScriptum S.R.L publishing group

120 High Road, East Finchley, London, N2 9ED, United Kingdom
Str. Armeneasca 28/1, office 1, Chisinau MD-2012, Republic of Moldova, Europe
Printed at: see last page
ISBN: 978-620-8-33659-2

BREASTFEEDING

AUTHORS:
MARIA CLARA SANTOS ARAÚJO ANTONIO DA COSTA CARDOSO NETO MÁRCIA SILVA DE OLIVEIRA

Breastfeeding is an instinctive and natural act, but it's also an art that you learn day by day.

(La Leche League)

SUMMARY

INTRODUCTION

Full maternal breastfeeding for up to six months is essential for the child's well-being in the early years, as recommended by the Ministry of Health (MoH). During the postpartum period, many women face significant challenges due to a lack of the necessary skills and knowledge. It is important that specialised professionals intervene in the prenatal period, during childbirth and in the postpartum period, with actions aimed at preventing, detecting and overcoming difficulties in mother-child interaction (Brasil, 2017).

The National Breastfeeding Policy in Brazil is supported by guidelines from the Ministry of Health that seek to "increase exclusive breastfeeding rates up to six months of age" (Brasil, 2017, p. 45). This policy also aims to integrate breastfeeding support actions into health, education and social assistance policies, promoting the creation of a favourable environment that ranges from training health professionals to ensuring appropriate spaces for breastfeeding in public and private environments.

The challenges to the effective implementation of this policy include improving the support infrastructure in hospitals and maternity wards and combating the influence of the breastmilk substitute industry. According to Santos, "the continuity of education and support for mothers, especially after hospital discharge, is crucial" to ensure the success of prolonged breastfeeding (Santos, 2019, p.399).

In this context, nursing care plays a key role in supporting breastfeeding. Trained nurses can provide valuable guidance and emotional support to mothers, helping to overcome common barriers to breastfeeding, such as latch-on difficulties, pain during breastfeeding and worries about breastfeeding. milk production. Early and continuous intervention by these professionals can improve exclusive and prolonged breastfeeding rates, promoting long-term health benefits for the child and the mother (Zanlorenzi et al., 2022).

Against this backdrop, this study seeks to answer the following guiding question: What are the benefits of nursing care for breastfeeding? The review will look at studies that demonstrate the effectiveness of nurse-led breastfeeding support programmes, as well as identifying successful strategies and challenges faced in practice.

The study seeks to evaluate nursing interventions and their impact on breastfeeding, with the aim of expanding knowledge about breast anatomy and physiology. This research provides an essential scientific foundation, enriching the academic field and serving as a teaching resource for the professionals involved.

The justification for carrying out this research is based on the need to address and overcome the challenges encountered during breastfeeding, providing an opportunity to implement more effective practices and continuous support for mothers. Nursing care is essential to guide and train mothers in correct breastfeeding technique, proper baby positioning and manipulation to avoid problems such as engorgement and fissures.In addition, the theoretical foundation will cover the anatomy and physiology of the mammary glands, detailing their structural composition, vascularisation and lymphatic drainage. It will explore hormonal regulation, highlighting the role of oestrogen, progesterone, prolactin and oxytocin in development and lactation. It will also analyse anatomical and physiological variations over the course of the menstrual cycle, pregnancy, lactation and menopause, as well as pathological such as mastitis, fibroadenomas and breast cancer, emphasising the importance of this knowledge for clinical practice and support for breastfeeding. This research will make relevant contributions by deepening our understanding of the importance of nursing care in breastfeeding. breastfeeding.

Through an detailed analysing of nursing interventions, it is hoped to elucidate the positive effects of these practices on the promotion and maintenance of breastfeeding. In addition, research into the anatomy and physiology of the mammary glands will provide a solid scientific basis, enabling nursing professionals to analyse the anatomy and physiology of the mammary glands.to offer more qualified support to mothers.

OBJECTIVES

GENERAL OBJECTIVE

Carry out a systematic review on the benefits of nursing care for breastfeeding.

SPECIFIC OBJECTIVES

Present breast anatomy and physiology and their characteristic aspects.
Identify the benefits of breastfeeding on the health of the child.

child.

To understand the importance ofnursing care in supporting breastfeeding.

THEORETICAL BACKGROUND

BREAST ANATOMY AND PHYSIOLOGY

The mammary glands are essential both for the nutrition of newborn babies and for a woman's general health. They are made up of different types of tissue that fulfil specific functions. Firstly, the outermost layer is made up of the skin, where the areola is located, a pigmented area that surrounds the nipple. The areola contains Montgomery's glands, which secrete a lubricating substance that is essential for breastfeeding (Biswas et al., 2022).

Describing it in detail, the authors emphasise: Mammary glands are compound, branched tubuloalveolar structures and a defining feature of mammals. Mammary glands evolved from epidermal apocrine glands, located on the ventral surface of the body. Mammary glands produce milk as a source of nutrition to support postnatal offspring survival and reproductive success in all mammals (Biswas et al., 2022, p.[1]).

Internally, the breast is made up of glandular tissue, adipose tissue and connective tissue. The glandular tissue is responsible for milk production and is organised into lobes and lobules, connected by lactiferous ducts that converge at the nipple. Adipose tissue gives the breast volume and shape, while connective tissue provides structural support (Rezende, 2019). In addition, the vascularisation of the mammary glands is mainly provided by the internal and lateral mammary arteries, ensuring adequate tissue nutrition. At the same time, the lymphatic system, made up of a network of vessels and lymph nodes, plays a decisive role in lymphatic drainage, preventing infections and facilitating the immune response (Biswas et al., 2022).

According to Pinho (2017), to ensure a complete understanding of the anatomical structure, it is vital to consider the variations that occur during the menstrual cycle, pregnancy and lactation, influenced by hormonal changes. In this context, the physiology of the mammary glands is regulated by a complex hormonal system that coordinates development and lactating function. During puberty, the increase in oestrogen and progesterone levels promotes the growth of mammary structures, preparing them for potential milk production in the future (Pinho, 2017; Viégas, 2019). During pregnancy, the hormones prolactin and oxytocin are essential. Prolactin stimulates milk production by the alveolar cells, while oxytocin promotes contraction of the lactiferous ducts, allowing milk to be ejected. This mechanism is fundamental for effective breastfeeding (Carreiro et al., 2018).

Consequently, the interaction between hormones and specific receptors in breast tissue results in dynamic changes, especially during the lactation and postpartum periods. This knowledge is essential for health professionals working in obstetrics and gynaecology, as it directly influences maternal and child care practices (Carreiro et al., 2018; Viégas, 2019). On the other hand, Rezende (2019) states that breasts have a variety of characteristics that vary between women, influenced by genetic, hormonal and environmental factors. Size, the shape and density of breast tissue are individualised aspects that can affect both function and aesthetics.In this sense, breast sensitivity is another important characteristic, varying throughout the menstrual cycle due to hormonal fluctuations. During pregnancy and lactation, sensitivity can increase significantly, reflecting the physiological changes that occur during these periods (Rezende, 2019; Pinho, 2017).

In contrast, it is essential to consider the pathological variations that can occur in the mammary glands, such as mastitis, fibroadenomas and breast cancer. Therefore, in-depth knowledge of mammary anatomy and physiology is relevant for the early detection and effective treatment of these conditions (Biswas et al., 2022).

Breast development throughout life

From birth, the breasts undergo continuous development, which intensifies during puberty. During childhood, the breasts remain in a latent state until the hormonal signals of puberty trigger the growth of the glandular and ductal tissues. This process is mainly influenced by the increase in oestrogen levels, which promotes the development of the lactiferous ducts and the growth of adipose tissue, resulting in the formation of the adult characteristics of the breast (Heijer; Blok; Dijkman, 2021).During adolescence, the breasts continue to develop, reaching functional and structural maturity. This period is marked by significant hormonal changes, which not only promote growth, but also the differentiation of breast tissue. Therefore, the authors further emphasise that: "Breast development during puberty is mediated by exposure to oestrogen, resulting in changes in both the volume and structure of breast tissue." (Heijer; Blok; Dijkman, 2021, p.2199, my translation).[2]
In this context, it is noted that: In healthy adult women, each breast has between 10 and 20 lactiferous units made up of secretory cells and ducts. These units are called lobules, which are arranged in the breast like the spokes of a wheel, with the areola and the nipple at their centre. The glandular portion is made up of alveoli which, joined together in the form of clusters, end in ducts. These unite to form larger ducts which, below the areola, dilate to form the lactiferous sinuses, which have the function of storing milk. The lactiferous sinuses narrow and flow into the

nipple (Rezende, 2019, p.231).

With the arrival of the menopause, there are significant changes in the structure and function of the breasts. The reduction in oestrogen and progesterone levels results in atrophy of the glandular tissue, which is progressively replaced by adipose and connective tissue. These changes can lead to a decrease in breast volume and firmness, as well as increasing susceptibility to certain pathological conditions, such as chronic mastitis and neoplasms (Rezende, 2019).

Functional aspects of lactation

Lactogenesis, the process of milk production, takes place in two distinct phases. The first begins during pregnancy, preparing the breasts for milk production. However, the second begins immediately after giving birth, triggered by a drop in progesterone levels and an increase in prolactin, resulting in the active production and secretion of milk (Silva; Janzen, 2023).

The authors go on to detail: Lactogenesis is a mechanism that occurs physiologically throughout pregnancy and continues in the puerperium. Lactogenesis II (or lactation) takes place between the second and third postpartum day, triggering lactation (Silva; Janzen, 2023, p.707). The baby's sucking is essential for the continued production of milk. The sucking action stimulates the nerves in the areola and nipple, sending signals to the brain to release oxytocin. This hormone promotes the contraction of the myoepithelial cells around the alveoli, ejecting the milk through the lactiferous ducts to the nipple. This mechanism ensures that milk is available for the newborn during breastfeeding (Rezende, 2019).

"All the studies have shown that sucking is associated with the release of oxytocin. [...] The correlation between milk production and the number of oxytocin pulses is of particular interest, as each oxytocin peak is linked to milk ejection." (Uvnäs-Moberg et al., 2020, p.30, my translation):[3] Thus, Chatterton et al. (2018) comments that continuous milk production is dependent on the baby's demand. The frequency and effectiveness of breastfeeding directly influences prolactin levels and, consequently, the amount of milk produced. Prolonged interruptions in breastfeeding can lead to reduced milk production, while frequent and efficient breastfeeding maintains lactation at adequate levels.

Breast health and pathologies

Mastitis is an inflammation of the breast, often associated with lactation. Caused by bacterial infections or blockages in the lactiferous ducts, mastitis presents symptoms such as pain, swelling, redness and fever (Uvnäs-Moberg et al., 2020). Treatment includes antibiotics, painkillers and measures to ensure continued breastfeeding, such as hand milking or the use of breast pumps (Sales et al., 2019).

The authors write in detail:

The best treatment is massage, followed by milking, application of local heat and/or cold, increased fluid intake and rest. [...] The most suitable antibiotics are penicillinase-resistant penicillins or cephalosporins, which cover betalactamase-producing Staphylococcus aureus, the most prevalent bacterium in mastitis cases (Sales et al., 2019, p.627).

Benign breast conditions such as cysts and fibroadenomas are common and generally pose no health risk, but they can cause discomfort and anxiety. Early detection and regular monitoring are essential to ensure that these conditions do not develop into more serious problems. Thus: "Benign breast lumps account for up to 80 per cent of palpable masses.

Fibroadenoma is the most common breast neoplasm in patients under 35 and cysts are more frequent in the perimenopause." (Nazário; Rego; Oliveira, 2017, p.211).However, scholars also report that breast cancer is one of the most common neoplasms among women. Early detection, through imaging tests such as mammograms and MRI scans, is crucial for effective treatment. Treatment options range from conservative surgeries to complete mastectomies, often combined with chemotherapy, radiotherapy and hormonal therapies (Nazário; Rego; Oliveira, 2017, p.211).

BREASTFEEDING: DEVELOPMENT VITAMIN

Lactation begins in the alveoli of the mammary glands, covering around two thirds of the breast structure. Milk is transported from the alveoli to the nipple via the lactiferous sinuses. Although oestrogen and progesterone are crucial for the physical development of the breasts during pregnancy, they prevent milky secretion. Prolactin, on the other hand, stimulates its production (Órfão; Gouvéia, 2023).

The anterior pituitary gland in mothers secretes prolactin, the concentration of which gradually increases from the fifth week of pregnancy until labour. This hormone plays a crucial role in the development and function of the mammary alveoli. During pregnancy, the placenta also secretes human chorionic somatomammotropin, a lactogenic hormone that supports maternal prolactin activity. Despite being present throughout pregnancy, the levels of these two hormones do not increase significantly due to the suppression caused by high levels of progesterone and oestrogen (Carvalho; Tamez, 2019). After the delivery process, the levels of the final two hormones are reduced, resulting in an increase in the placenta's lactogen and prolactin levels, which then initiates milk production. Milk production is sustained as long as the baby suckles on the nipples, as the act of suckling causes the hypothalamus to release prolactin-releasing factor and maintain prolactin levels, which is responsible for milk production (Carvalho; Tamez, 2019).

Breastfeeding is considered the most ideal method of providing nutrition to newborn babies. It is a decisive stage that generates countless benefits for the health of both mother and child, which in turn has a positive impact on society in general. The act of breastfeeding not only provides nutrition, but also creates a deep bodily connection that has emotional and biological significance for the mother-child bond. In addition, breastfeeding can influence the mother's physical and mental well-being (Leite, 2023).

Despite the plethora of scientific evidence confirming the superiority of breastfeeding compared to other infant feeding methods, and the efforts of national and international organisations to educate and inform mothers about the critical importance of exclusive breastfeeding, the number of mothers who exclusively breastfeed their infants remains below the recommended level (Brazil, 2018).

In order to change these statistics, health professionals play a key role. This approach must recognise the mother as the central figure in the breastfeeding process, and must involve valuing her, listening to her and developing essential skills (Brazil, 2018).

Breast milk is widely considered to be a comprehensive source of nutrition, full of essential nutrients that can meet all of a baby's needs in the first six months of life. As the child grows from six to nine months, breast milk is able to provide three quarters of the proteins needed. Even beyond this stage, it still serves as an excellent protein supplement for a balanced diet. In addition to protein, breast milk also contains vital minerals, vitamins, fats and sugars (Leite, 2023).During the first few days after birth, the milk produced by the mother's breasts is called colostrum. This milk is rich in antibodies, leucocytes and vitamin A, and has a laxative effect on the infant, by helping to eliminate meconium, a pasty, greenish substance that is excreted during the newborn's first bowel movements. In doing so, colostrum prevents jaundice. Colostrum is generated from the first to the seventh day postpartum, and is known as mature milk from the eighth to the fifteenth day. Both colostrum and mature milk work together to supplement the child's immune system against childhood infections (Lima, 2017).

Understanding and mastering the definitions of the breastfeeding process, recognised by the World Health Organisation (WHO) and respected worldwide, is of great importance. Exclusive breastfeeding - when the child receives only breast milk, straight from the breast or milked, or human milk from another source, with no other liquids or solids, with the exception of drops or syrups containing vitamins, oral rehydration salts, mineral supplements or medicines. Predominant breastfeeding - when the child receives, in addition to breast milk, water or water-based drinks (sweetened water, teas, infusions), fruit juices and ritual fluids. Breastfeeding - when the child receives breast milk (straight from the breast or milked), regardless of whether or not they receive other foods. Supplemented breastfeeding

- when the child receives, in addition to breast milk, any solid or semi-solid food with the aim of complementing it, not replacing it. In this category, the child may receive another type of milk in addition to breast milk, but this is not considered complementary food. Mixed or partial breastfeeding - when the child receives breast milk and other types of milk (Brazil, 2018, p.12). When babies are exclusively breastfed for the first six months of life, it has been shown that they gain twice as much weight

at birth. Breast milk continues to have the advantage of being an economical source of food for infants, as well as eliminating the risk of contamination by harmful microorganisms that can be found in formula milk, formula and bottles. In addition, it is the which also supports the baby's healthy development and growth (Souza, 2019).
Breastfeeding offers several advantages for mums, such as protection against breast cancer, preventing conception and increasing the emotional connection between mother and child. There are also additional benefits for the family as a whole, including a reduction in financial costs, as there is no need to buy food for the baby during this period. In addition, a well-nourished and breastfed child is less likely to fall ill and require hospitalisation, leading to a better quality of life and greater harmony in the home (Brazil, 2018).

Benefits of breastfeeding

Breast milk is widely recognised as the ideal food for newborn babies, as it has a balanced combination of essential nutrients, including proteins, fats, carbohydrates, vitamins and minerals. Its composition adapts to the baby's nutritional needs as they grow, ensuring an adequate supply at all stages of development. In addition, human milk is easily digested and absorbed by the newborn's immature digestive system, preventing problems such as colic and constipation (Pellegrine et al., 2018). The benefits of breastfeeding go beyond nutrition. Colostrum, the first milk produced by the mother, is particularly rich in proteins, immunoglobulins and growth factors, providing immediate protection against infections and promoting the maturation of the digestive tract (Silva; Janzen, 2023). One of the most outstanding aspects of breastfeeding is its ability to strengthen the baby's immune system. Human milk contains antibodies, leucocytes and other bioactive substances that help protect the newborn against a wide range of bacterial, viral and parasitic infections. The presence of secretory immunoglobulin "A" (IgA) in human milk forms a protective layer on the mucous membranes of the gastrointestinal and respiratory tracts, preventing the adhesion and invasion of pathogens (Pellegrine et al., 2018; Uvnäs-Moberg et al., 2020). In this scenario, breast milk promotes the development of a healthy gut microbiota, which is essential for long-term immunity. Studies have shown that breastfed babies have a lower incidence of infectious diseases, such as otitis media, diarrhoea, respiratory and urinary infections, compared to those who are formula-fed. artificial formulas (Palheta; Aguiar, 2021).

Palheta and Aguiar (2021) report that breastfeeding is also associated with cognitive benefits, because the long-chain polyunsaturated fatty acids, especially docosahexaenoic acid (DHA) present in human milk, are important for brain development and vision.

Despite the nutrients, the act of breastfeeding strengthens the mother-baby bond, providing a safe and stimulating environment that favours emotional and cognitive development. Interaction during breastfeeding stimulates the release of hormones such as oxytocin, which promotes attachment and neuropsychological development (Macedo et al., 2022; Sardinha et al., 2019).

Breastfeeding is associated with a significant reduction in the risk of various chronic diseases throughout life. Epidemiological studies suggest that breastfed babies are less likely to develop obesity, type 1 and type 2 diabetes, hypertension and diseases in adulthood. The mechanisms proposed for these protective effects include the regulation of energy metabolism, the formation of healthy eating habits and metabolic programming induced by the bioactive components of human milk

(Zanlorenzi et al., 2022). Furthermore, exclusive breastfeeding in the first six months of life is associated with a lower risk of developing allergies and autoimmune diseases such as asthma and coeliac disease. This immunomodulatory effect is attributed to the immunological factors present in breast milk and the promotion of a balanced intestinal microbiota (Macedo et al., 2022). In addition to the physical and immunological benefits, breastfeeding offers psychosocial advantages for both the baby and the mother. Skin-to-skin contact during breastfeeding strengthens the emotional bond and provides comfort and security for the newborn. This bond is essential for emotional socialdevelopment ofthe child, contributing to the formation of a secure and healthy attachment (Sardinha et al., 2019). For the mother, breastfeeding provides a sense of fulfilment and connection with the baby, as well as mental health benefits. The release of oxytocin during breastfeeding promotes relaxation and reduces the risk of postpartum depression. In addition, breastfeeding helps the mother to regain her pre-pregnancy weight more quickly and reduces the risk of breast and ovarian cancer (Zanlorenzi et al., 2022).

BREASTFEEDING: NURSING CARE

There is a great deal of information about breastfeeding available to women; however, just knowing the benefits of breastfeeding is not enough to keep them doing it. In order to maintain breastfeeding, women often need professional assistance to offer them the support they need (Carvalho; Tames, 2019).

To ensure that women receive the best possible care, nursing plays a vital role, and it is essential that its actions are informed by current scientific knowledge to promote preventive measures against early weaning and low milk production (Lima, 2017).The role of the nursing professional is to provide comprehensive care to the puerperal woman. With this knowledge, they can help in more complex situations, thus avoiding premature abandonment of breastfeeding. It is essential to be adequately prepared and equipped to deal with any challenges that may arise and to have a plan for each obstacle to avoid early weaning, as described by Lima (2017).

Initiating breastfeeding education in the early stages of pregnancy is a crucial task for health professionals. It is important to provide pregnant couples with access to literature, educational resources and qualified counsellors who can offer adequate guidance during this period. Sufficient information should be provided to the pregnant woman and her partner so that they can make an informed decision about the ideal method of feeding their child (Carvalho; Tamez, 2019). When it comes to a healthy breastfeeding practice, it's important for nurses to be able to clearly guide pregnant women on the importance of maintaining a nutritious diet. In order to offer comprehensive and empathetic support, it is essential to address each women with respect and help them overcome their fears, obstacles or uncertainties (Athanázio et al. 2013).The Ministry of Health requires nurses to possess not only fundamental knowledge and proficiency in breastfeeding, but also the ability to communicate effectively and unambiguously with postpartum women. The technique of breastfeeding counselling serves as an excellent way of achieving this goal. This approach is characterised by an emphasis on facilitating informed decision-making on the part of the mother. It involves actively listening to her concerns, empathising with her needs and carefully weighing up the pros and cons of various options, rather than just prescribing a course of action (Brazil, 2018).

The literature by Carvalho and Tamez (2019) outlines the necessary steps for successful counselling. The basic principles of counselling should include: Active listening (listening first, observing, asking questions, assessing the knowledge or information that the woman and her partner have); Body language (using eye-to-eye contact without barriers, showing respect, patience in listening, counselling in a private setting); Attention and empathy (taking into account the couple's feelings, answering questions without making judgements); Decision-making (identifying the source of the couple's misinformation, offering timely information related to the situation, guiding them to make the best decision). "Follow-up (being involved in the nursing mother's process, being available to see her again, identifying with the couple the journey that has taken place, and being prepared to support their decisions)." (Carvalho; Tamez, 2019, p.122).

In this sense, caring for nursing mothers who visit a primary health care unit is a fundamental responsibility of nursing professionals, who must have a differentiated approach that enables them to guide these mothers in preventing early weaning and in (Athanázio et al. 2013).

During the initial antenatal appointment, routine laboratory tests, a complete physical examination and a thorough history are usually carried out. This interview should include a breast examination, which can help reassure the mother that her breasts are normal and, if there are any problems, the best treatment options can be recommended, giving the mother enough time to prepare for breastfeeding (Athanázio et al. 2013; Carvalho; Tamez, 2019).

The consultation should be carried out by a group made up of a nurse and an obstetrician, avoiding redundant questions and assessments. It is important to emphasise that the group should provide information materials that illustrate the short- and long-term benefits of breastfeeding for both mother and child (Carvalho; Tamez, 2019).

In pregnancy monitoring, educational initiatives such as theoretical and practical guidance are often employed. To ensure maximum participation, it is recommended that timetables be thoroughly researched. A group size of 12 to 16 participants is ideal, as it allows for a non-oppressive environment. Demonstrations, including the use of dolls, are often used to teach breastfeeding techniques, correct latch-on and positions (Athanázio et al. 2013).

The postpartum period, or puerperium, is a phase in which: The establishment of rules that encourage breastfeeding immediately after birth, while still in the delivery or recovery room, has been shown to positively influence the incidence of breastfeeding, as well as its duration." In the puerperium, rooming-in is recommended, where the baby is constantly in the company of the mother and has access to the breast on demand, without strict breastfeeding schedules, which promotes increased milk production and avoids the use of supplementation, as well as beneficial psychological factors such as the promotion of mother-child attachment. The first step in assisting a breastfeeding mother is to assess how she feels about it. The decision to breastfeed or not should have already been made in the prenatal period, a factor that predisposes the mother to whether or not she will succeed in breastfeeding after giving birth. Mothers are best helped by professionals who demonstrate that breastfeeding is the natural way to feed their child (Carvalho; Tamez, 2019, p. 124). Establishing a relationship of trust with the mother is a crucial aspect of the nurse's role. This involves boosting her self-esteem and confidence to enable her to care for her baby independently. At the beginning of each shift, the nurse should assess the mother to determine the appropriate nursing care plan for breastfeeding. The information obtained during the hospital visit can be used for future comparisons or in the event of breastfeeding complications (Leite, 2023).

According to Carvalho and Tamez, the recommendations are: Breast examination to check the milk supply and prevent any problems that may arise. Assessing the newborn's general condition, helping the mother to understand their behaviour and how to respond to their needs. Include the father and/or support person in the assessment and teaching of breastfeeding, as they have become an important support for the mother. Review specific breastfeeding techniques with the couple, emphasise care during breastfeeding once at home; remind parents that breastfeeding depends on the balance between milk production and breast emptying and on the infant's ability to suck. Provide a guide on how to detect problems and how to intervene, factors that will be the key to optimal milk production, reflected in the baby's normal growth. Being present during the first breastfeeding session in order to assess and answer questions that arise (Carvalho; Tamez, 2019, p. 125).

It is also recommended that mothers take various precautions during the breastfeeding period after giving birth, including maintaining a nutrient-rich and balanced diet, avoiding any unapproved medication In addition, mothers should ask their doctor to refrain from applying creams to the areola of the breast, consume plenty of fluids and manually remove any ointment if there are cracks in the teat before breastfeeding to help the baby latch on more easily. In addition, mums should wear suitable bras and take care when positioning the baby to feed, ensuring that they suck enough milk (Leite, 2023).

METHODLOGY

This is a systematic study carried out with the aim of producing a review of the benefits of nursing care for breastfeeding.

This study used the following databases: MEDLINE (Medical Literature Analysis and Retrieval System Online), BNDEF (Database of Clinical Pharmacological Studies) and LILACS (Latin American and Caribbean Literature on Health Sciences).

To facilitate access to the database searches, the BVS (Biblioteca Virtual de Sade) regional portal was used. The descriptors were chosen according to DeCS (Health Sciences Descriptors) and MeSH (Medical Subject Headings). In accordance with the DeCS and MeSH list, the terms used were: "Nursing care, Breastfeeding and Infant". In addition to the descriptors, the Boolean operators "AND" and "OR" were used to combine the terms in the databases.

It followed the recommendations of the PRISMA declaration, which consists of a checklist of 27 elements and a flow chart, to help authors improve the communication of the review (Moher et al., 2009; Urrútia; Bonfill, 2010). The data for this study was collected from the databases between February and May 2024, with the aim of answering the following guiding question: What are the benefits of nursing care for breastfeeding? According to the databases consulted, a total of 7,400 articles were identified, distributed as follows: 3,000 articles in MEDLINE, 2,900 articles in LILACS and 1,500 articles in BDENF. Initially, 4,800 articles were discarded due to the filters applied: availability of full text, language - Portuguese and publication period between 2019 and 2024.

Thus, 2,600 articles were selected after this filtering. Subsequently, 800 duplicate articles were eliminated, leaving 1,800 articles. Of these, 1,760 articles were excluded after analysing the title and abstract, resulting in the selection of 40 full articles for eligibility assessment. Of these, 26 articles were discarded because they did not meet the study's objective, resulting in 14 final articles included in the research, as detailed in the flow diagram of the scientific article selection process. What stands out in the current study is the author's interpretation and personal critical analysis that led to the inclusion of the articles for the study. The author chose materials with information that appropriately considered the study as presented here and that met his expectations.

The inclusion criteria were original articles published in Portuguese in the previous five years, which addressed the topic to be studied and allowed full access to the study content. Non-inclusion criteria were articles eliminated by filters, incomplete articles published before 2019, duplicate articles, articles excluded bytitle abstract that did not meet the study objective, complete articles were excluded from the analysis after careful reading that were not available in full. To collect the data, key words were initially selected to search for articles with content that covered the subject of this study. While the data was being collected from the databases, a flow chart was constructed to clarify how it was carried out.

to select the articles included in the study. In order to analyse the data, a composite table was drawn up identifying the authors, the year the work was published and the title of the article, database, shows, relevant results. The results were interpreted and analysed based on a synthesis of the results comparing the data found in the articles included in this study. See the flowchart below:

Figure 1 - Flow diagram of the scientific article selection process

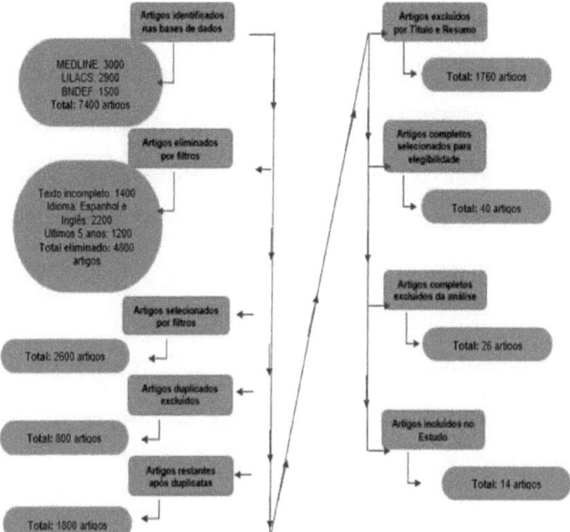

RESULTS AND DISCUSSIONS

The results obtained through this systematic review enrich our understanding of the anatomical and physiological complexity of the mammary glands, emphasising their fundamental importance in the lactation process. This understanding is essential for clinical practice in areas such as obstetrics and gynaecology, as it deepens knowledge of the biological bases that support breastfeeding. The analysis of the data collected was meticulously supported by a selection of recent and relevant scientific studies, which contribute significantly to elucidating the individual variations and patterns associated with breastfeeding. Integrating this data with existing literature is crucial to ensure a holistic and up-to-date understanding. In order to clearly and systematically present the findings of this review, the following is a table that correlates the observed data with the reference studies in the field. The table not only makes it easier to visualise the information, but also allows for a direct comparison with pre-existing data in scientific literature:

Table 1 - Articles used in the systematic review

NO.	Author / Year	Title / Base data	Method / Show	Relevant results
01	Anjos; Almeida; Picanço / 2022.	Nurses' perceptions of o Breastfeeding in the immediate puerperium / BDENF.	A descriptive, exploratory, qualitative field study with 13 nurses from a public maternity hospital in Salvador, Bahia. in Salvador, Bahia.	The study reports the identification of fissures and breast engorgement as the main complications. continuous counselling from prenatal care through to the puerperium was highlighted as crucial. The study also found that the benefits of breastfeeding facilitated counselling, while the high workload was a hindrance.

Continued from Table 1 - Articles used in the systematic review

NO.	Author / Year	Title / Base data	Method / Show	Relevant results
02	Camargo et al. / 2024.	Early breastfeeding injuries / LILACS.	Retrospective, cross-sectional study using primary data and a database of photographic images of two randomised clinical trials. Evaluation of 115 breastfeeding and186 images photographs.	In the study, the findings refer to moderate nipple pain in breastfeeding women and the presence of nipple lesions with more than 25% of the nipple surface area affected. It was also observed that pain during breastfeeding was moderate and the lesions significantly affected more than 25% of the nipple surface.
03	Cunha et al. / 2024.	Factors associated with breastfeeding breastfeeding birth in maternity hospitals linked to the Stork Network, Brazil, 2016-2017 / MEDLINE.	Cross-sectional study with data from Second evaluation cycle 2016-2017 of the Stork Network, covering the whole of Brazil.	The data found in the study show that the prevalence of breastfeeding in the first hour was 31 per cent, and in the 24 hours, 96.6 per cent. Factors that increased the chances of breastfeeding in the first hour included the presence of a companion during hospitalisation, skin-to-skin contact, vaginal delivery, nurse-led birth care and accreditation of the unit in the Baby-Friendly Hospital Initiative. Similar results were observed at 24 hours, with an additional association with maternal age under the age of 20.

Continued from Table 1 - Articles used in the systematic review

NO.	Author / Year	Title / Database	Method / Show	Relevant results
04	Melo et al. / 2023	Breastfeeding: prevalence and conditioning factors in a city in the interior of the Zona da Mata region of Minas Gerais / LILACS	A descriptive, quantitative cross-sectional study involving 118 women.	The findings show that 56.7% of the interviewees did not know the term "Exclusive Breastfeeding" at the time of the interview. It was noted that 23.7 per cent thought that there are situations in which the baby should not be not be breastfed. Only 19.4 per cent reported believing in the existence of "weak milk", while 100% recognised breast milk as a suitable food for babies. the baby.
05	Martins et al. / 2024.	Breastfeeding breastfeeding clinic care as an important action to promote breastfeeding / MEDLINE.	Report of experience implemented in a health centre in Belo Horizonte, August 2019. Sample of 204 breastfeeding women attended from August 2018 to January 2021.	The study reports that the clinic assisted 204 breastfeeding women with average age of 33 years. 50 per cent of the breastfeeding women had completed high school and the average family income was up to two minimum wages. It was also observed that the majority of breastfeeding women (75%) were multiparous. Around 53.9 per cent of puerperal women reported difficulties in breastfeeding, mainly related to a pain and problems with the breastfeeding.

Continued from Table 1 - Articles used in the systematic review

NO.	Author / Year	Title / Database	Method/ Show	Relevant results
06	Macedo et al. / 2022.	Assimilation of puerperal women on educational practices on breastfeeding duringprenatal care/ BDENF.	Exploratory, qualitative study with19 puerperal women in rooming-ina public hospital.	The study found that the puerperal women were on average 26 years old, with a predominance of prenatal care in the public sector. It was also observed that the majority wanted to breastfeed, but there was a lack of health education activities on breastfeeding during prenatal care.
07	Iopp; Massafera ; De Bortoli / 2023.	A role of nurses in promoting, encouraging e management/ MEDLINE.	Cross-sectional, descriptive, quantitative study carried out in Pato Branco, involving 13 primary care nurses. primary care.	The findings show that the majority of UBSs do not have written rules on breastfeeding (92.3%), do not implement breastfeeding support groups (69.2%) and do not involve family members in support actions (76.9%). It was also observed that the main complications attended to were nipple cracks, difficulty in latching on and breastfeeding. grip and breast engorgement.
08	Hirano; Baggio; Ferrari / 2021.	Breastfeeding and complementary feeding: mothers' experiencese health professionals in a border region / BDENF.	Research exploratory-descriptive, qualitative study with 12 mothers (5 foreign) and12 health professionals (8 nurses, 2 doctors, 2 nutritionists) in Foz do Iguaçu, PR.	The study states that the average The average age of the mothers was 27.8 years, most of whom were married and primiparous. As for the professionals, the average age was 36.5 years. 92.3% of the professionals reported a lack of written rules on breastfeeding. It was also observed that the challenges included high workloads, a lack of multi-professional teams and inadequate flow of care for foreign and foreign-born children. brasiguayas.

Continued from Table 1 - Articles used in the systematic review

NO.	Author / Year	Title / Database	Method / Show	Relevant results
09	Mosquera etal./ 2023.	Prevalence e Predictors of breastfeeding in the MINA-Brazil / MEDLINE.	Study of cohort with 1.143 mother-child pairs registered in the Maternal and Child cohort cohort in Acre (MINA-Brazil).	The findings show that the frequency of exclusive breastfeeding (EBF) at 3 and 6 months was 33 per cent and 10.8 per cent, respectively. Factors such as primiparity, pre-milk feeding and dummy use in the first week of life were predictors of early cessation of EBF. It was observed that the duration of breastfeeding and continued breastfeeding (BF) were lower than those of children who were not breastfed. WHO recommendations.
10	Moreira et al. / 2021.	Management counselling as an instrument for improving indices of exclusive breastfeeding: an integrative review	Qualitative integrative review with 21 articles selected from 757 found in the Scielo, PubMed, Lilacs, Cinahl and VHL.	It was observed that the review showed that not receiving information about breastfeeding during prenatal care interferes with maintaining exclusive breastfeeding. breastfeeding. Supportive practices and directive counselling had a positive impact on maintaining exclusive breastfeeding. Exclusive breastfeeding.
11	Rodrigues et al. / 2021.	Challenges faced by primiparous women the breastfeeding process / LILACS.	Descriptive, exploratory and qualitative character with 20 lactating primiparas.	The findings of this study show that 65 per cent of mothers reported breast pain, 40 per cent had cracks, 35 per cent found it difficult to hold the baby, and 30 per cent felt insecure about milk production. Professional and family support was considered essential for successful breastfeeding.

Continued from Table 1 - Articles used in the systematic review

NO.	Author / Year	Title / Database	Method / Show	Relevant results
12	Silva et al. / 2021.	Experience e Attitudes about breastfeeding breastfeeding / LILACS.	Qualitative study mediated action research with 12 pregnant women in two UBS in Cajazeiras, PB.	The study found that 75 per cent of pregnant women were aware of the benefits of breastfeeding for the mother-child binomial, but 50 per cent were unaware of the benefits for the mother. 60 per cent reported that their motivation to breastfeed was still influenced by local myths and beliefs, leading to weaning early.
13	Santos et al. / 2023.	Difficulties with breastfeeding and feeding practices / MEDLINE.	Cross-sectional, descriptive study with 96 mothers attending a public maternity hospital in Rio de Janeiro.	The study found that 64 per cent of mothers reported difficulties breastfeeding, including pain (45 per cent), nipple cracks (30 per cent) and insecurity about the amount of milk (25 per cent). Professional support was crucial in overcoming difficulties and maintaining breastfeeding exclusive.
14	Santos et al. / 2024.	Breastfeeding at discharge and at third stage of the Kangaroo Method among hospitalised preterm newborns / MEDLINE.	Longitudinal, retrospective study with 186 neonates (<37 weeks) admitted to the to the NICU in 2018 and 2019.	The study found that the rate of exclusive breastfeeding (EBF) was 73.1 per cent at hospital discharge, 74 per cent at first return and 68.1 per cent at last return. Younger mothers with higher education and neonates with higher birth weights who received exclusive human milk during hospitalisation had a higher rate of exclusive breastfeeding. greater likelihood of SMA.

Source: Author (2024).

The studies analysed highlight different perspectives on breastfeeding practices and challenges, from nurses' perceptions to the conditioning factors that influence breastfeeding.breastfeeding. By comparing the results of these studies, it is possible to identify patterns and discrepancies that reflect the complexity of breastfeeding dynamics in different Brazilian contexts.According to research by Anjos, Almeida and Picanço (2022), which identifies fissures and breast engorgement as the main complications in the immediate puerperium, emphasising continuous guidance as a crucial tool for mitigating these problems.

Continuous education from prenatal to postpartum emerges as a focal point for preventing complications, a view shared by Macedo et al. (2022), who point out the scarcity of educational activities on breastfeeding during prenatal care. This lack of preparation can contribute to the difficulties faced by puerperal women who, although they want to breastfeed, are often deprived of practical information.

In addition, Camargo et al. (2024) document the prevalence of nipple lesions, with more than 25% of the nipple surface affected, correlating these lesions with moderate nipple pain during breastfeeding. These data suggest a pressing need for more effective interventions in pain management and injury prevention, a point that dialogues with Martins et al.'s (2024) practical approach in the breastfeeding clinic. Additionally, in the outpatient clinic, 53.9% of breastfeeding women reported difficulties with breastfeeding, mainly related to pain and inadequate technique, reinforcing the importance of specialised centres that provide direct and personalised support to breastfeeding women. Cunha et al. (2024) detailed in their study that the prevalence of breastfeeding immediately after birth is only 31 per cent, a considerably low rate. However, there is evidence of an increase The study found a substantial improvement in this proportion, reaching 96.6 per cent in the first 24 hours of the newborn's life. The study identifies several factors that contribute to this improvement, including the presence of a companion during labour, the establishment of skin-to-skin contact between mother and child soon after birth, vaginal delivery and the support of specialised maternity nurses.These elements are seen as crucial to promoting breastfeeding in the first hours of life. However, the research suggests that appropriate hospital practices and specialised training for health professionals are essential to facilitate the initiation of breastfeeding, underlining the importance of institutional policies and training that prioritise these conditions. Melo et al. (2023) show a great lack of information about Exclusive Breastfeeding, with 56.7% of the women interviewed confessing to being completely unaware of this terminology. In addition, the survey found that 19.4 per cent of the participants reported believing in the "weak milk" myth. This reflects the difficulties imposed by misconceptions and misinformation, which are serious obstacles to proper and effective breastfeeding.These results underline the urgent need for educational programmes and information campaigns that can demystify these misconceptions and promote greater understanding of the benefits and procedures of exclusive breastfeeding. From this perspective, Iopp, Massafera and Bortoli (2023) enrich the discussion by examining the infrastructure and institutional policies in force in Basic Health Units (BHUs). The authors highlight the lack of formalised guidelines on breastfeeding in primary healthcare units. 92.3 per cent of UBS, and 69.2 per cent of these units do not implement support groups for this practice. This lack of an established policy, as well as the absence of support groups, is identified as a considerable obstacle for health professionals, as well as for breastfeeding women, who often need these resources to deal with the difficulties inherent in the breastfeeding process. The lack of these institutional instruments jeopardises the effectiveness of actions to promote and support breastfeeding, reflecting a gap in the care offered to women during this critical phase. On the other hand, the research carried out by Hirano, Baggio and Ferrari (2021) in the city of Foz do Iguaçu reveals a worrying lack of written regulations relating to breastfeeding among 92.3 per cent of health workers, which highlights a significant deficiency in current institutional policies. This normative gap is particularly critical in a region characterised by its vast cultural diversity, where the implementation of more robust and well-defined policies could potentially substantially improve the support offered to mothers.The absence of these guidelines jeopardises the quality of care provided, as well as limiting the ability of health professionals to provide adequate guidance and support, adapted to the cultural and social specificities of the population they serve. Therefore, correcting this flaw in institutional policies is an urgent necessity for improving maternal and child care in contexts of great diversity.This lack of policies is directly reflected in the operational obstacles and uniformity of the service, analogous to the problems reported in urban environments by Santos et al. (2023), where the lack lack of support and correct information results in high incidences of breastfeeding problems, such as pain and nipple cracks, experienced by 64 per cent of mothers.However, according to the findings of the MINA-Brazil cohort study carried out by Mosquera et al. (2023), a worrying reality was found in which only 33 per cent of mothers manage to maintain exclusive breastfeeding until their baby is three months old. This percentage drops sharply to just 10.8 per cent at six months. These figures reveal a significant challenge when it comes to promoting and sustaining exclusive breastfeeding, highlighting the need for more effective public policies and interventions to support mothers in this process over time.The sharp drop in exclusive breastfeeding rates over the first six months underlines the importance of a multidimensional approach that involves both strengthening support networks and practising educational and care strategies aimed at continuing breastfeeding, which is essential for children's health and development.

The comparative analysis of these data with the results obtained by Moreira et al. (2021) highlights the critical importance of prenatal counselling in promoting breastfeeding. The lack of clear and specific guidance during this period contributes directly to the early interruption of breastfeeding, in addition to factors such as primiparity and the use of dummies, which have been identified as predictors of the early termination of exclusive breastfeeding.Research by Moreira et al. (2021) revealed that mothers who did not receive prenatal counselling were substantially more likely to stop exclusive breastfeeding before the six months recommended by health guidelines. These The findings underline the need for health policies that strengthen education and support during the gestational period in order to ensure better breastfeeding rates and, consequently, promote infant health and well-being.According to the study carried out by Rodrigues et al. (2021), which investigated primiparous mothers facing various physical and psychological challenges in the breastfeeding process, the results converge with the findings of Silva et al. (2021), who emphasise the influence of regional myths and beliefs on decisions related to breastfeeding. Both studies emphasise that insufficient support, both informational and affective, contributes to the adoption of inadequate breastfeeding practices, highlighting a critical area where adequate guidance and support could make a substantial difference.

Rodrigues et al. (2021) reported that 65 per cent of primiparous mothers experienced significant pain during breastfeeding, and 40 per cent of them suffered from breast fissures, factors that can discourage continued breastfeeding. These data underline the urgent need for interventions aimed at strengthening support for mothers in order to reduce the obstacles that hinder the practice of exclusive breastfeeding and thus promote better maternal and child health outcomes.Similarly, the longitudinal analysis carried out by Santos et al. (2024) on premature neonates reveals that, despite the additional challenges faced by this population, exclusive breastfeeding rates remain remarkably high. This success is attributed to the intensive nutritional and educational support offered during the hospitalisation period. Specifically, the exclusive breastfeeding rate was 73.1 per cent at the time of hospital discharge, increased slightly to 74 per cent on the first return and, although it fell slightly, still remained at 68.1 per cent on the last return. This scenario contrasts with the conditions described in other studies, where a lack of adequate support and misinformation result in substantially lower rates of exclusive breastfeeding. The research by Santos et al. (2024) highlights the importance of well-structured and continuous interventions to ensure the success of breastfeeding, even in situations involving additional complications such as prematurity.Through these comparisons, it becomes clear that uniformity in the implementation of support policies, accurate breastfeeding education and the availability of resources for mothers in a variety of contexts are essential to raising breastfeeding rates. In light of the above, the interconnections between the studies suggest that, regardless of the geographical or socio-economic context, strengthening professional and family support, together with transparent policies and well-structured institutional regulations, could mitigate many of the challenges faced by mothers during the lactation period.

CONCLUSION

This topic enabled an in-depth analysis of the complexity and importance of the mammary glands in lactation, as well as the fundamental role of nursing care in breastfeeding. The specific objectives, aimed at evaluating the benefits of this assistance and elucidating breast anatomy and physiology, were fully achieved, offering a detailed overview of the structures involved and the physiological mechanisms of lactation. Likewise, the frequent challenges faced by mothers during the breastfeeding period were identified. It has become clear that breastfeeding goes beyond simple infant nutrition, establishing itself as a crucial factor for healthy infant development and maternal well-being, emphasising the need for specialised and continuous support during this period. Training and constant support for health professionals, especially nurses, appear to be essential components in fostering an efficient and prolonged breastfeeding practice.The research also emphasised the crucial role of public health policies and continuous professional development as essential strategies for improving exclusive and extended breastfeeding rates. The conclusions emphasise the urgency of individualised approaches to breastfeeding care, taking into account the singularities of each situation. In response to the guiding question, "What are the benefits of nursing care for breastfeeding?", this study validated that nursing support not only facilitates the practice of breastfeeding, but also mitigates the usual complications during this process, providing a more comfortable experience. breastfeeding is more rewarding and effective for both mum and baby. Suggestions for future research include longitudinal studies that can monitor the effects of educational actions aimed at health professionals on breastfeeding practices in different socio-cultural contexts. It would also be valuable to explore the long-term impact of nursing support for breastfeeding on maternal and child health in deprived communities, where there is often limited access to adequate health services. This study highlights the urgent need for a more comprehensive health policy and educational projects that address the complexity of breastfeeding, taking into account the particular needs of each mother and baby, with the aim of optimising breastfeeding practices and promoting the health and well-being of the mother-child duo.

REFERENCES

ANJOS, C. R.; ALMEIDA, C. S.; PICANÇO, C. M. Nurses' perception of breastfeeding in the immediate puerperium. **Rev baiana enferm**, 2022, v. 36, p. e43626. Available at: http://www.revenf.bvs.br/pdf/rbaen/v36/2178-8650-rbaen-36-e43626.pdf. Accessed on: 25 June 2024.

ATHANÁZIO, A. R. et al. The Importance of Nurses in Encouraging Breastfeeding to Newborns: Integrative Review. **Revista de enfermagem UFPE online**, pp. 4119-4129, 2013. Available at: https://periodicos.ufpe.br/revistas/revistaenfermagem/article/view/11640/13725. Accessed on: 29 May 2023.

BISWAS, S. K.; BANERJEE, S.; BAKER, G. W.; KUO, C.-Y.; CHOWDHURY, I. The mammary gland: basic structure and molecular signalling during development. **International Journal of Molecular Sciences**, v. 23, n. 7, p. 3883, 2022. Available in em:https://www.mdpi.com/1422-0067/23/7/3883. Accessed on: 25 May 2024.

BRAZIL. **Ministry of Health**. National Breastfeeding Policy. Brasília, DF, 2017.

BRAZIL. Ministry of Health. **Breastfeeding, Distribution of Infant Milks and Formulas in Health Establishments and Legislation**. 2. ed. Brasília/DF 2018.

CAMARGO, B. T. S.; SAÑUDO, A.; KUSAHARA, D. M.; COCA, K. P. Injuries early breastfeeding: analysis of photographic images and clinical associations. **Rev Bras Enferm**, 2024, v. 77, n. 1, p.1-8. Available at: https://www.scielo.br/j/reben/a/FysXq63dG5ZQffTdDLCSfCP/?lang=pt&for

mat=pdf. Accessed on: 25 June 2024.

CARREIRO, J. A.; FRANCISCO, A. A.; ABRÃO, A. C. F. V.; MARCACINE, K. O.;
ABUCHAIN, E. S. V.; COCA, K. P. Difficulties related to breastfeeding: an analysis of a specialised breastfeeding service. **Acta paul. Enferm [online]**. 2018, vol. 31, n. 4, pp. 430-438. Available at:<https://www.scielo.br/j/ape/a/VpgWq MNCRFF5vLVJvFfPSXz/?lang=en&format=pdf>. Accessed on: 26 May 2024.

CARVALHO, M. R.; TAMEZ, R. N. **Amamentação:** Bases cientificas. 2 ed. Rio de Janeiro: Guanabara Koogan, 2019. pp 07, 18.

CHATTERTON, R. T.; HILL, P. D.; ALDAG, J. C.; HODGES, K. R.; BELKNAP, S. M.;
ZINAMAN, M. J. Relationship of plasma concentrations of oxytocin and prolactin with milk production in mothers of preterm infants: influence of stress. **The Journal of Clinical Endocrinology & Metabolism**, 2018, v.85, n.10, p. 3661-3668. Available at:https://doi.org/10.1210/jcem.85.10.6912. Accessed on: 26 May 2024.

CUNHA, J. F.; GAMA, S. G. N.; THOMAZ, E. B. A. F.; GOMES, M. A. S. M.; AYRES,
B. V. S.; SILVA, C. M. F. P.; LEAL, M. C.; BITTENCOURT, S. D. A. **Cien Saude Colet**,2024, v. 29, p. e04332023. Available in:

https://www.scielo.br/j/csc/a/pCqVNhycB5n8LtbhQ8kP7fc/?lang=pt&format=pdf. Accessed on: 25 June 2024.

HEIJER, M.; BLOK, C. J. M.; DIJKMAN, B. A. M.; Sustained Breast Development and Breast Anthropometric Changes in 3 Years of Gender-Affirming Hormone Treatment. **The Journal of Clinical Endocrinology & Metabolism**, v. 106, n. 2, p. e782-e790, 2021. Available at: https://academic.oup.com/jcem/article/98/6/2198/2536872. Accessed on:

26 May 2024.

HIRANO, A. R.; BAGGIO, M. A.; FERRARI, R. A. Breastfeeding and complementary feeding: experiences of mothers and health professionals in a border region. **Enferm Foco**, 2021, v. 12, n. 6, p. 1132-1138. Available at: http://revista.cofen.gov.br/index.php/enfermagem/article/view/4787/1287. Accessed on: 25 June 2024.

IOPP, P. H.; MASSAFERA, G. I.; BORTOLI, C. F. C. The role of nurses in promoting, encouraging and managing breastfeeding. **Enferm Foco**, 2023, v. 14, p. 1-6. Disponível em: https://enfermfoco.org/wp-content/uploads/articles_xml/2357- 707X-enfoco-14-e-202344/2357-707X-enfoco-14-e-202344.pdf. Accessed on: 25 June 2024.

LEITE, S. M. M. **Breastfeeding and the factors that interfere in the initial phase. Monograph presented to the State University of Paraíba-UEPB**, pp. 01-38, 2023. Available at: <http://dspace.bc.uepb.edu.br/jspui/bitstream/12345 6789/929/1/PDF%20%20S%C3%A9rgio%20Mafra%20de%20Moura%20 Leite.pdf> Accessed on: 29 May 2023.

LIMA, S. S. **The benefit of breastfeeding:** mother-child binomial. Monograph presented to the Anhanguera de Campo Grande Institution, pp.01-31, 2017.

MACEDO, D. C. F. S.; CARVALHO, J. S. N.; OLIVEIRA, J. S. B.; LIMA, L. S. V.; SUTO,C. S. S.; HAIMENIS, R. P. Assimilation of puerperal women on educational practices on breastfeeding during prenatal care. **Rev baiana enferm**, 2022, v. 26, p. 1-11. Available at: http://www.revenf.bvs.br/pdf/rbaen/v36/2178-8650-rbaen-36-e46765.pdf. Accessed on: 25 June 2024.

MARTINS, C. D.; BICALHO, C. V.; FURLAN, R. M. M.; FRICHE, A. A. L.; MOTTA, A.R. Breastfeeding clinic in primary care as an important action to promote breastfeeding: an experience report. **CoDAS**, 2024, v. 36, n. 3,p.1-6.Available at: https://www.scielo.br/j/codas/a/QbgxqGjKj6SZBpc8dhCQ5Yd/?lang=pt&format=pdf. Accessed on: 25 June 2024.

MELO, L. B. L.; SILVA, L. N.; SOUZA, M. L. P.; ANDRADE, M. A. C.; FÓFANO, G. A.
Breastfeeding: prevalence and conditioning factors in a city in the interior of the Zona da Mata region of Minas Gerais. **Revista Científica da Escola Estadual de Saúde Pública de Goiás "Cândido Santiago"**, 2023, v. 9, n. 9b1, p. 1-14. Available at: https://www.revista.esap.go.gov.br/index.php/resap/article/view/490/279. Accessed on: 25 June 2024.

MOHER, D., LIBERATI, A., TETZLAFF, J., ALTMAN, D.G., & PRISMA Group. Preferred reporting items for systematic reviews and meta-analyses: the PRISMA statement. **PLoS Medicine**, v.6, n.7, e1000097, 2009.

MOREIRA, M. A.; FILIPIN, M. A. G.; ARAÚJO JUNIOR, J. C.; NASCIMENTO, P. S.;
MARQUES, P. F.; RIBEIRO, P. S. Directive counselling as a tool for improving exclusive breastfeeding rates: an integrative review. **Revista Nursing**, 2021, v. 24, n. 281, p. 6552-6560. Available at: https://revistanursing.com.br/index.php/revistanursing/article/view/2011/2459. Accessed on: 25 June 2024.

MOSQUERA, P. S.; LOURENÇO, B. H.; MATIJASEVICH, A.; CASTRO, M. C.;CARDOSO, M. A. Prevalence and predictors of breastfeeding in the MINA-Brazil cohort. **Revista de Saúde Pública**, 2023, v. 57, supl. 2, p. 1-13. Available at: https://www.scielo.br/j/rsp/a/ydWR6RT8JPVKPsVP3k9vNhC/?lang=pt&for

mat=pdf.Accessed on: 25 June 2024.

NAZÁRIO, A. C. P.; REGO, M. F.; OLIVEIRA, V. M. Benign breast nodules: a review of differential diagnoses and management. **Revista Brasileira de Ginecologia e Obstetrícia**, v. 29, n. 4, p. 211-219, 2017. Available at:< https://www.scielo.br/j/rbgo/a/WNYzrcNtfVfCYWhRnCpT45m/?lang=pt&format=pdf>. Accessed on: 26 May 2024.

ÓRFÃO, A.; GOUVEIA, C. Anatomy and physiology of lactation. **Revista Portuguesa de Clínica Geral**, v. 25, p. 347-354, 2023. Available at: http://www.rpmgf.pt/ojs/index.php/rpmgf/article/view/10631. Accessed on: 29 May 2023.

PALHETA, Q. A. F.; AGUIAR, M. de F. R. Importância da assistência de enfermagem para a promoção do aleitamento materno. **Acervo Saúde**, São Paulo, v. 8, n. 1, p. 1- 10, Jan./2021. Available at: https://acervomais.com.br/index.php/enfermagem/article/view/5926. Accessed on: 29 May 2023.

PELLEGRINE, J. B.; KOOPMANS, F. F.; PESSANHA, H. L.; RUFINO, C. G.; FARIAS,H. P. S. Popular health education: human milk donation in a community in Rio de Janeiro, Brazil. **Interface**, v. 18, supl. 2, p. 1499-1506, 2018.

PINHO, A. L. N. Prevention and treatment of breast fissures based on scientific evidence: an integrative literature review. **Revista Brasileira de Saúde Materno-Infantil**, v. 14, n. 3, p. 325-338, 2017. Available at: https://ares.unasus.gov.br/acervo/html/ARES/4765/1/3259.pdf. Accessed on: 25 May 2024.

RESENDE, M. A. Natural breastfeeding: aids for the nursing team part I. **Revista da Escola de Enfermagem da USP**, São Paulo, v. 23, n. 3, p. 231-242, dec. 2019. Available at:

https://www.scielo.br/j/reeusp/a/LQQtgHWJ9BFh5ScdgfL
QhKD/?format=pdf. Accessed on: 25 May 2023.

RODRIGUES, G. M. M.; FERREIRA, E. S.; NERI, D. T.; RODRIGUES, D. P.; FARIAS,
J. R.; ARAÚJO, Y. I. S. Challenges presented by primiparous women in the breastfeeding process. **Revista Nursing (Brazilian Edition, Print)**, v. 24, n. 281, p. 6270-6279, Oct. 2021. vailable at: https://www.revistanursing.com.br/index.php/revistanursing/article/view/19
65/2387. Accessed on: 25 June 2024.

SALES, A. N.; VIEIRA, G. O.; MOURA, M. S. Q.; ALMEIDA, S. P. T. M. A.; VIEIRA, T.
O. Puerperal mastitis: a study of predisposing factors. **RBGO**, v. 22, n. 10, 2019. Available at:
https://www.scielo.br/j/rbgo/a/XfGzhQSKnpKdPK5XnC4VyWM/?lang
=en&format=pdf. Accessed on: 26 May 2024.

SARDINHA, D. M.; MACIEL, D. O.; GOUVEIA, S. C.; PAMPLONA, F. C.; SARDINHA,L. M.; CARVALHO, M. S. B.; SILVA, A. G. I. Promotion of breastfeeding in prenatal care by nurses. **Revista de Enfermagem UFPE online**, Recife,v.13, n.3,p. 852-857,Mar.2019.Available at: https://periodicos.ufpe.br/revistas/index.php/revistaenfermagem/article/vie
w/238361/ 31593. Accessed on: 26 May 2024.

SANTOS, M. T. Challenges to the implementation of breastfeeding policy in Brazil. **Revista Brasileira de Saúde Materno Infantil**, Recife, v. 19, n. 2, p. 395-402, 2019. Available at:
https://www.scielo.br/j/rbsmi/a/7GpKkZ3LsN9Nm3sP9HbJpNp/?lang=pt.
Accessed on: 25 June 2024.

SANTOS, A. C. S .; CARMONA, E. V.; SANFELICE, C. F. O.; MAFETONI, R. R.;LOPES, M. H. B. M.; BALAMINUT, T. Breastfeeding at discharge and in the third stage of the Kangaroo Method among hospitalised premature newborns. **Rev Esc Enferm**. USP, 2024, v. 00, p. 1-11. Available at: https://doi.org/10.1590/1980 - 220XREEUSP-2023-0383pt. Accessed on: 25 June 2024.

SANTOS, B. O. M. F.; SILVA, M. D. B.; DIAS, B. A. S.; ALVES, D. S. B.; MELO, E. C.P. Difficulties with breastfeeding and feeding practices. **Revista Enfermagem UERJ**, Rio de Janeiro, 2023, v. 31, p. 1- 8. Available at: https://www.e-publicacoes.uerj.br/enfermagemuerj/article/view/73485/47853. Accessed on: 25 June 2024.

SILVA, A. B. L.; ALVES, B. P.; SÁ, B. A.; SOUZA, J. W. R.; ANDRADE, M. E.;FERNANDES, M. C. Experience and attitudes of pregnant women about breastfeeding. **Rev Bras Promoç Saúde**, 2021, v. 34, p. 1-9. Available at: https://ojs.unifor.br/RBPS/article/view/11903/pdf. Accessed on: 25 June 2024.

SILVA, B. C.; JANZEN, D. C. Risk factors associated with delayed lactogenesis II: literature review. **Enfermagem Brasil**, v. 22, n. 5, p. 707-720, 2023. Available at:<https://convergenceseditorial.com.br/index.php/enfermagembrasil/article/view/ 5266/8793>. Accessed on: 26 May 2024.

SOUZA, S. N.D.H. Breastfeeding from the perspective of programme vulnerability and care. **Cad. Saúde Pública**, Rio de Janeiro, v.29 n.6, p.1186- 1194, jun, 2019. Available at: <http://www.scielo.br/pdf/csp/v29n6/a15v29n6.pdf>.Accessed on: 23 May 2023.

URRÚTIA, G.; BONFILL, X. PRISMA statement: a proposal to improve the publication of systematic reviews and metaanalyses. **Med Clin (Barc),** v.135, n.11, p.507-511, 2010.

UVNÄS-MOBERG, K.; EKSTRÖM-BERGSTRÖM, A.; BUCKLEY, S.; MASSAROTTI, C.; PAJALIC, Z.; LUEGMAIR, K.; KOTLOWSKA, A.;

LENGLER, L.; OLZA, I.; GRYLKA-BAESCHLIN, S .; LEAHY-WARREN, P .; HADJIGEORGIOU, E .;
VILLARMEA, S. Maternal plasma levels of oxytocin during breastfeeding - A systematic review. **Plos One**, v. 15, n. 8, e0235806, 2020. Available at: https://doi.org/10.1371/journal.pone.0235806. Accessed on: 26 May 2024.

VIÉGAS, C. M. P. Topographical anatomy x treatment plans. **Journal of Radiotherapy e Oncology**,v.7,n.2,p.78-92.2019.Available at: https://www.inca.gov.br/sites/ufu.sti.inca.local/files/media/document/seminario- radiotherapy-chapter-two-breast-part-2.pdf. Accessed on: 25 May 2024.

ZANLORENZI, G. B.; WALL, M. L.; ALDRIGHI, J. D.; BENEDET, D. C. F.; SKUPIEN,S. V.; SOUZA, S. R. R. K. Fragilities and potentialities of nursing care in breastfeeding in primary care: an integrative review. **Revista de Enfermagem da UFSM**, v. 12, e36, 9 Aug. 2022. Available at: https://doi.org/10.5902/2179769268253. Accessed on: 25 May 2024.

AUTHORS' BIOGRAPHIES

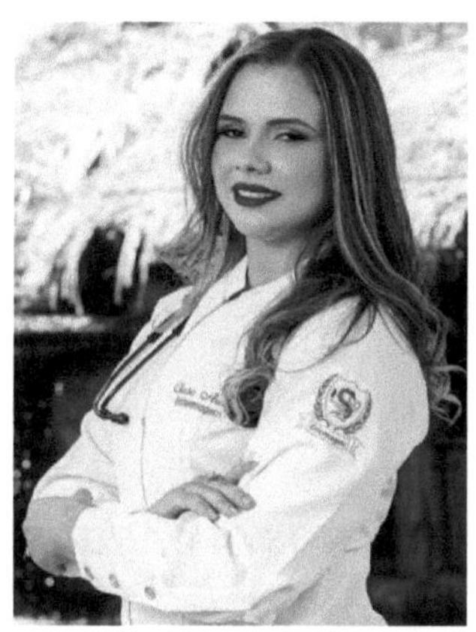

MARIA CLARA SANTOS ARAÚJO

Bachelor's Degree in Nursing from Santa Luzia College-FSL. Nursing Technician from the Santa Luzia Technical School of Commerce. Expertise in Primary Care. Research in health.

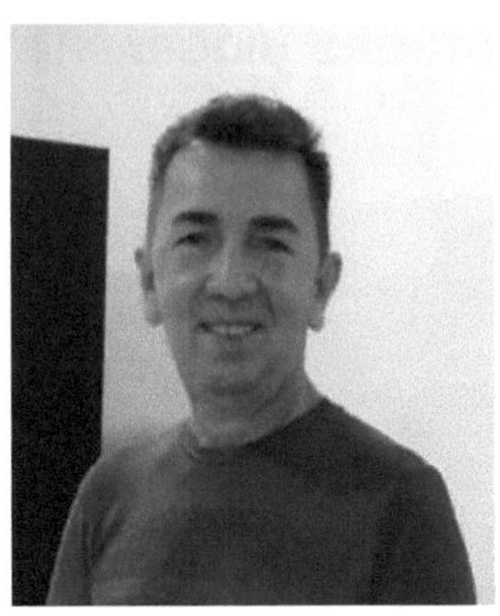

ANTONIO DA COSTA CARDOSO NETO

Post-Doctorate in Psychology from the University of Flores - Buenos Aires / Argentina (2023). PhD in Collective Health from the Federal University of Maranhão - UFMA (2021). PhD in Public Health Sciences from the University of Business and Social Sciences - UCES, Buenos Aires / Argentina (2018). Specialist in School Administration from the Cândido Mendes University, Rio de Janeiro (2010). Specialist in Elderly Health from the Estácio de Sá University, Rio de Janeiro (2011). Graduated in Bachelor's Nursing from the Universidade CEUMA / MA (2008). Graduated in Pedagogy from the State University of Maranhão - UEMA (2001). He is the Coordinator of Postgraduate Research and Extension, Professor of Scientific Methodology and Member of the Structuring Teaching Centre of the Nursing course at Faculdade Santa Luzia -FSL (2017 - current), a teacher of Basic Education in the public education network of the Municipality of Santa Inês/Maranhão (1998 - current). He has been Coordinator of the Undergraduate Nursing Course since its creation (2012-2018), Academic Director (2018-2023), Institutional Prosecutor (PI) (2017-2023) and Institutional Researcher -CENSUP (2018) at Faculdade Santa Luzia - FSL. He was a coordinator and teacher of technical courses at the Santa

Luzia Technical School of Commerce (ETCSL) / Maranhão (1996- 2021). 2017). Assistant researcher at the Federal University of Maranhão - UFMA (2006-2008). Researcher and Principal Sponsor of the Project: Biopsychosocial Education and Quality of Life for the Elderly. He has experience in drawing up Pedagogical Projects for Undergraduate Courses and drawing up Institutional Development Plans (PDI) Contact: (098) 981090921. E-mail: cardosoneto.acc@gmail.com; cardosonetofsl2018@outlook.com.br. ORCID: https://orcid.org/0000-0003-3771-2821

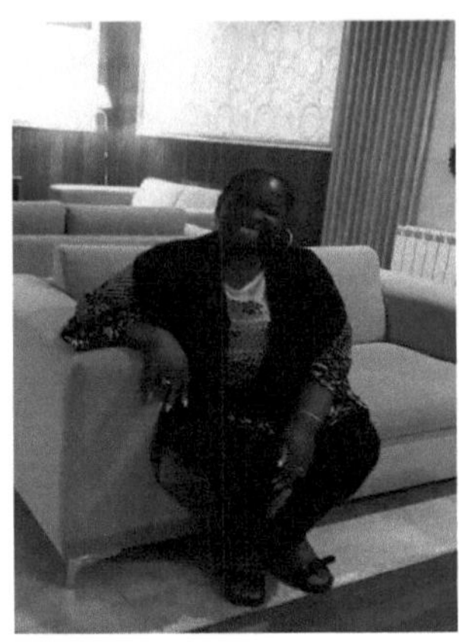

MARCIA SILVA DE OLIVEIRA

Post-Doctorate in Psychology - University of Flores (UFLO), Argentina. PhD in Public Health Sciences - Universidad de Ciencias Empresariales y Sociales (UCES), Argentina. Collaborating researcher at CITAB - Centre for Research and Agro-environmental and Biological Technologies at the University of Trás-os-Montes and Alto Douro/Portugal. Master in Health Sciences - University of Brasília (UnB). Postgraduate in Clinical Analyses (Cytopathology) - São Judas Tadeu College/RJ. Postgraduate

Degree in Pathology - Castelo Branco University/RJ. Postgraduate in University Teaching (Research Methodology and Pedagogical Research and Practice) - UniCEUB/DF. Graduated in Biological Sciences - Medical Modality (Biomedicine) from the State University of Rio de Janeiro (Anatomy). General/Pedagogical Coordinator of the Brasília Campus of Universidade Paulista (UNIP/Brasília). Lecturer in Pathology, Immunology, Didactics Applied to Nursing, Educational Practice in Health and Integrating Seminar on the Nursing course at Faculdade Santa Lu zia (FSL)/Santa Inês/MA. Lecturer with experience in organising, participating in, coordinating, planning and monitoring health and education projects, both inside and outside pedagogical learning spaces. Good interpersonal relationships, responsibility and dedication to work activities. Biomedical Supervisor at Dr Maricondi Ltda Medical Laboratory (WAMA Diagnóstica), São Carlos/SP (Costa Verde Unit - Itaguaí/RJ). Lecturer in the subjects of Safety, Environment and Health and Quality Management System at the Foundation to Support the Technical School of the State of Rio de Janeiro (FAETEC/RJ) Lecturer on undergraduate courses in Medicine, Dentistry, Nursing, Veterinary Medicine and Architecture and Urbanism at the Faculdades Integradas do Planalto Central (FACIPLAC/DF). Lecturer on undergraduate courses in Biomedicine, Physiotherapy, Psychology, Biological Sciences and Mathematics at Universidade Pau lista (UNIP - Campus Brasília). Coordinator and lecturer on postgraduate and extension courses at the Evangelical Educational Institute of the Centre-West - UNIECO/DF. Lecturer in Hormonology on the Postgraduate course in Clinical, Toxicological and Bromatological Analyses at the Instituto Brasil Pesquisa e Extensão - IBEP. Full Researcher at the Centre for Health Promotion Studies and Inclusive Projects at the University of Brasilia - NESPROM/UnB.

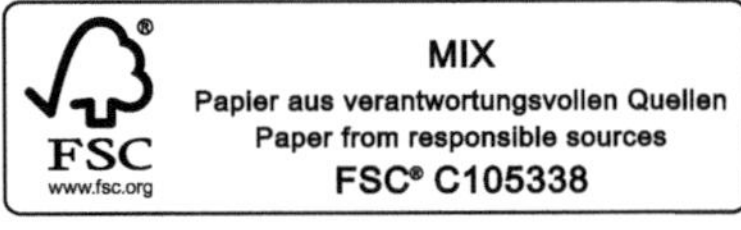

Printed by Books on Demand GmbH, Norderstedt / Germany